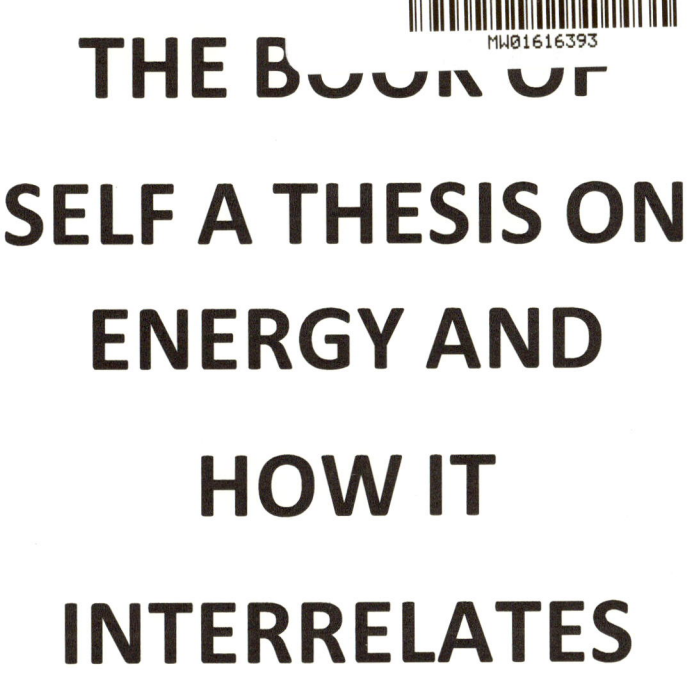

THE BOOK OF SELF A THESIS ON ENERGY AND HOW IT INTERRELATES

FLOYD WILLIAMS

NOTHING RESTS.EVERYTHING MOVES. EVERYTHING VIBRATES.

AFRICAN PROVERB

ACKNOWLEDGEMENTS

Thanks to the life source, universe, family, and friends. Much power to those in the belly of the beast criminal injustice system.

INTRODUCTION

Floyd Williams is an American Born revolutionary, author, and yogi, whose practice consists of kemetic yoga. Born and raised in Saint Paul Minnesota to parents, who believed in the power of knowledge, as well as, the might of the pen! The Book of Self A Thesis on Energy and How it Interrelates, is the author's fourth title. Other titles are: Unspoken Truth, The Origin of Racism, and The Holy Black Papyrus.

Floyd Williams is the type of man, who writes as he speaks; meaning he does not write unless he absolutely has something of value to say and give. The Book of Self A Thesis on Energy And How it Interrelates is a book, truly dedicated towards the revealing of man's full potential by unveiling his/her being to them by way of explaining our inter-connectedness to all energy and life on the planet, rather it be the heavens, earth, animals, or the atmosphere.

The author wants us to know we are way more, than hueman/human beings, we are energy beings; for human only defines pigmentation and, it only defines man being at a certain level of wisdom. The key to life and health is energy. When our pulse is taken, it is measuring energy, when a EKG is done, it is measuring energy. When our bodies are consuming food such as: chicken or broccoli it is not the chicken or broccoli, that is keeping us alive.

However, it is the unit of energy referred to as calories, which sustains us.

The more we as a people acknowledge the importance of energy and enhance our knowledge of it, the author believes our sense of self, as well as our quality of life will improve. These are a couple objectives of this monumental work. The Book of Self A Thesis on Energy And How it Interrelates is written in such a clear concise way, that it is empowering and rather a layman or a scholar, this read can be followed and gleaned from. The words and descriptions are so illustrative, that the imagery imposed upon the readers mind will seem, as if it is flowing from themselves.

THE BOOK OF SELF A THESIS ON ENERGY AND HOW IT INTERRELATES FLOYD WILLIAMS

As humans we are way more than, what the eyes behold. We are what I like to refer to as energy beings and have a direct relationship to the environment around us, below us, and above us. It is because of this, that we are bio-logical. We are biological beings. Bio, means relating to life and logical refers to our brains, minds, and the unique ability to use rationale; put simply the power of choice. The most sacred animating part of man is the unseen. This unseen part of man has the biggest influence upon us affecting human behavior.

Bio: a combining form meaning "life" occurring in loan words from Greek (biography); on this model, used in the formation of compound words. [Greek bios-life] [Latin, vivus, living]. (Webster's New Universal Unabridged Dictionary)

Logic: 1. The science that investigates the principles governing correct or reliable inference.2. a method of reasoning or argumentation. (Webster's New Universal Unabridged Dictionary)

The same life force, which sustains, as well as, animates what we observe on earth and admire above us is what animates us. So, therefore in certain cultures before they kill or remove, something from nature, they speak to it, "excuse me tree! But I need you for this purpose." One of the biggest signs we have in relation to our intimate connection attesting to the oneness of our beings is the oxygen, air, breath in the form of respiration, and it is that, which gives us life. So, in all the sacred texts revered by man, the physical or the silhouette of man does not come to being or alive, until the blowing of breath into. This life force is the same as the intangible elements around us, that is classified as gaseous viscous fluids, which pervades the atmosphere. Breath is energy and energy is breath and breath and energy equals spirit. Examine these words closely from the root. Breath comes from Greek word "brodem," meaning vapor, steam. And spirit comes from Latin word "Spiritus," and "spirare," meaning to breath.

All energy is one! The life force we take in as air is the medium, that allows us to feel as biological beings, to taste, to hear, to smell, to see. This medium of air is the highway, so to say of vibration. As above, so below. As within, so, it is without. Over 70% of the earth is covered by water. Over 70% of our bodies is composed of water. Our brains are 90% water; what does this mean for us? What is the significance of this relating to us? Water is the quintessence of life and origin of life. Sperm/semen/seamen; even the ovum is a kind of water and the embryo rests in water, in the womb. It is surrounded by water, and prior to birth the water is broke. Water acts as a cushion in the body surrounds the organs, the joints, and even the brain to aid in keeping in place and absorption of shock. Water deprivation pertinent to circulatory system of blood, will cause it to thicken, forcing

the heart to work harder to circulate the blood throughout the system.

In the scientific realm key part of blood is called hemoglobin. Hemoglobin produces the robust red color to blood, as it pulls from the sun. Very, important piece I want to point out is, that heme transfers the oxygen inside of our cells allowing for energy exchange. Remember, the oxygen is breath/spirit, and, if water is insufficient our bodies we can say, short circuits. Water, also, regulates temperature, removes waste. Through, this detailing I am trying to spell out the magical power of water and to convey, that water is 100% energy! And water is immortal, water is everlasting and indestructible. Just as energy does not die; it only transforms. Water can be liquid, solid(ice), precipitation, condensation, cloud forming; eventually coming back to earth in form of snow, rain, hail, or dew. Yet, it does not go away, just takes on another form. So, this makes water an excellent conductor of energy. So, this makes man an excellent conductor of energy, like the sky above; which we see displayed in the sky as lighting cuts across it. And through the spectrum of color's during sunset/sunrise.

How can I connect this to us through the maxim of as above, so below? As within, so without? Prime example being sometimes a person can come in contact with us and we may experience, what is known as a shock. We may get shocked; a shock like lightning is an electrical discharge. As human beings we have, what is called an aura (see chapter in my book The Holy Black Papyrus, Walking Lion the Aura Man), where the color spectrum can be viewed. The atmosphere around us is a womb. Out of the physical womb of our mother's, we are birthed and enter another womb, we identify, as the world, and through, this womb of the world as viable human beings we are nurtured. Along, with this, just as in the womb we have a physical umbilical cord, but, as viable human biological beings! Our umbilical cord is our "respiration," that is in truth is a variation of water, which carries vibration, frequencies, and this allows for us to feel and pick up the vibrations of the cosmos, planets, sun, and moon, based on energy running through us. Based on the tuning of the mind and I say tuning, because I equate the mind to a radio dial. So, this means based on thought we can fine tune and alter our energy, thus effecting and directing where it goes. Effecting its time and length of travel.

Our energy channel runs up the up spine in a criss crossing upwards motion and meeting at point in between the eye brows known as third eye and is emitted outwards projecting like a beam, and this electrical energy beam is never broken. It sends and receives, acting as a conduit. If, it was to break, then we could not receive. This criss

THE BOOK OF SELF A THESIS ON ENERGY AND HOW IT INTERRELATES FLOYD WILLIAMS

crossing motion of life force up the spine is where the symbolism of medical caduceus is taken from; it mirrors exactly the pattern of energy in our bodies. So far, a lot has been expounded on in relation to us energy beings. How we interconnect with it and are one with it; more adequately put extensions of energy, in all its various expressions composed of protons, electrons, and neutrons. For me as above, so below and as within, so without is a constant center of thought and a maxim I hold firmly to. Intimately visualizing my energy being functioning in the same exact manner, as the living organism, we refer to as the earth and the heavens above we admire.

Heavenly anatomy in relation to our anatomy, the earth has layers, as we do, which, is the lithosphere, asthenosphere, upper mantle, lower mantle, outer core, and inner core. Our layers are looked at as chakras; different vortexes of energy each with various frequencies, in relation to speed, determined by density; just as how, it is measured in organism of earth(seismology). Our inner core is our solar plexus and the organism the earth's core is a solar plexus. This inner core is a solid composed mainly of iron, outer core is a liquid; from this is generated, that, which is deemed as electromagnetism. How and why is this important? Excellent question!

Its importance lies in the protective energy field, that is created, it is this energy field, which, protects from cosmic storms, solar flares, in short, this protective energy field is the aura of the earth. Sounds familiar right? We have an aura and it operates in the same exact manner. The core of the earth is just as hot as the sun; so, its referred to as the solar plexus. Within our energy beings at the center of our solar plexus is a system of nerves connected to autonomic nervous system, parasympathetic/sympathetic with ganglion. This center sends or emits energy acting as a conduit portal. What I like to refer to as the ether-net of internet. We are surrounded by ether in our environment; this ether is a variant expression of energy, in which I see, it as being real powerful. I equate it to a black hole and connect to colors of aura, being interconnected and working in conjunction to mind (our thoughts). I see the ether field in a sense as a second self (but being our real self); so, to say, because it's wellness determines our aura. If it is weak our energy slows down too much, becoming heavy and in addition to that, as organic beings we become to open and susceptible to attacks of beings, that on the present low dense waves being emitted (recall role of earth's aura and apply to self). To make plain sound is a language, color is a language. Here is where our diet and minds come into play and why it is encouraged to eat a variety of colors of fruits and vegetables, because the seven primary colors taught in art, which are the colors of the rainbow, are one with us; inseparable from our bodies. Each food color carries a unique frequency merging and feeding colors of rainbow chakras, that pervade our

THE BOOK OF SELF A THESIS ON ENERGY AND HOW IT INTERRELATES FLOYD WILLIAMS

energy beings. Consequently, affecting our etheric bodies and aura.

It is my thought, that the cerebrospinal fluid is a primordial fluid of old. How old cannot be estimated, yet, I would estimate it to be older, than the 4.5-billion-year-old earth. And it contains the building blocks of life carbon, melanin, proteins, it is an immortal fluid responsible for healing, regeneration. I deem the cerebrospinal fluid to be a viscous ether and ether to be an airy cerebrospinal fluid. As a people we are truly one with the cosmos and the organism of the earth. We are only a variant expression of it, and one with the energy responsible for it all. We are only extensions of energy.

THE BOOK OF SELF A THESIS ON ENERGY AND HOW IT INTERRELATES FLOYD WILLIAMS

WE ARE THE WI-FI AND WHY THE ESTABLISHMENT DON'T WANT US INTUNE WITH IT

Whatever, it is that man utilizes and has invented, all comes from the human blueprint of man, the blueprint of nature. The human blueprint of man and nature references, how everything is patterned and mimicked off nature, rather it be in in shape, function or how energy moves interrelating with us. As I present myself to you through these pages I have one primary focus I will be elaborating on, which I judge to be of utmost importance in our journey of mental, spiritual liberation, out of which, has become infamously known as the matrix. I did not include the physical in our journey of liberation; for one it cannot be separated from our being and once the mind and spirit is liberated, then naturally the physical will follow. Thus, the saying as popularized by Envogue "free your mind and the rest will follow.)

We are organic energy beings full of energy. Protons, electrons, and neutrons, constantly flow through us, in us, and around us. Technology has come on the scene and in recent years, man has done some phenomenal things with it. Great advances have been and are being made in computer Technology. As intriguing and wonderful as the computer is; its wonder and intrigue does not surpass, that of the first computer. What is the first computer? And no! It was not created by IBM. The first computer is the brain, which, typically composes 2% of our body weight and varies according to race. Yes! The first computer is the brain and the brain consist of an intricate networking system of cables/nerves, that make up the central nervous system or neuro immune system connecting to spinal cord. The brain is the source of mind and the brain generates electrical impulses emitting waves. Does this make you think of anything? As I continue to expound, it will all hit home within the next few sentences.

By energy flowing in us and emittance of energy, which sends information and receives information, also being foundation of formation of imagination, it forms mental images we see. So, this is a type of intangible monitor/screen; from this we should see, that we possess a wireless anatomy and from this the internet was mimicked and patterned. Between 1983-1990 was the internet cultivated and created. However, the internet has in truth been around since time immemorial, since man first set foot on the planet. The biggest feature of the internet besides being able to communicate and performance of tasks, is the capability of the system commonly known as wi-fi, which is captured in the title of this chapter.

Our natural wi-fi as a people is what is number one in life. Our natural wi-fi is, what we must protect as a people and is what is under attack! As well as what the so-called powers that be or what the establishment does not, want us connected to. Everything they do is designed to keep our connection to our wi-fi severed, through primarily ensuring; for one, that as a people we have no cognition of it. The purpose of this is to keep from real potential and to secure the establishment's government rulership. Keep in mind, that the first computer is the brain and the brain with other glands a part of the brain connected to it such as: pineal gland and pituitary gland emits waves. These waves are energy waves, which enhances life experiences, enhances the being, and connects to the cosmos. Therefore, meditation is of importance, why prayer is of importance, why spirituality is of importance.

It's a divine communication system. So, we are dealing with a language. What is the language? It's the language of freedom, liberation, autonomy, and free thought. And all of this reflects the spirit, the so-called establishment does not want you to have! Why, is this? Because, if this is allowed, then they (establishment) cannot rule, if they do not possess your mind. When you possess the mind, you possess and control the spirit. To make clearer, our natural wi-fi can be viewed as our intuition our intuition is akin to the mind in a sense, because, it is a subtle communication system an intangible energy field network. The intuition has a strong premonition and all too often we suppress the intuition which is always 100% right. We suppress and reject, even though we internally agree with it, but, due to

THE BOOK OF SELF A THESIS ON ENERGY AND
HOW IT INTERRELATES FLOYD WILLIAMS

programming and conditioning we accept opposite of
what intuition is telling us and we accept what
establishment says and its false standards of morality, law,
and what we think is intelligence. We go against, what we
know, for it! So, I believe the picture is now clear; so, I say
protect and embrace your wi-fi and as you do we shall see
change across the planet and the people will have their
power back.

SIDE NOTE- I WROTE THIS WRITING A WHILE AGO AND IT
HAS BEEN GROWING INSIDE ME FOR YEARS. BUT JUST AS I
BEGAN THE PROCESS OF TYPING THIS BOOK. THE TRUMP
ADMINISTRATION IS PUSHING WHAT IS CALLED "NET
NETURALITY." WAKE UP PEOPLE FAST!

✓   THE ORIGIN OF RACISM

✓   UNSPOKEN TRUTH

✓   THE HOLY BLACK PAPYRUS

✓ THE BOOK OF
SELF A THESIS ON
ENERGY AND
HOW IT
INTERRELATES

TITLES CAN BE FOUND ON

✓ LULU.COM

✓ AMAZON.COM

AUTHOR'S CONTACT INFORMATION

✓TWITTER
@FLOYDWILLIAMS14

✓FACEBOOK
FLOYDWILLIAMS/14

✓E-MAIL
FLOYDWILLIAMS14@GMAIL
.COM

KEY WORDS AND TERMS

✓ **ENERGY**

✓ **INTERRELATES**

✓ **VIBRATION**

✓ **UNIVERSE IN LATIN UNI, ONE VERTERE, TURN**

- ✓ BEING

- ✓ POTENTIAL

- ✓ CALORIE IN FRENCH IS CALORE, HEAT

- ✓ INTER-CONNECTEDNESS

- ✓ HUE MEANS COLOR MAN REPRESENTS A DEGREE

- ✓ MELANIN

- ✓ CARBON

- ✓ DARK MATTER THE POTENTIAL OF ENERGY

- ✓ ETHER

- ✓ BIOLOGICAL

- ✓ ORGANISM

- ✓ RESPIRATION

- ✓ SPIRIT

- ✓ OXYGEN

- ✓ BREATH

- ✓ PHOTOSYNTHESIS

- ✓ ATMOSPHERE

- ✓ PROTONS

- ✓ ELECTRONS

- ✓ NEUTRONS

- ✓ CHAKRAS

- ✓ COSMOS

- ✓ AURA

- ✓ NERVOUS SYSTEM

- ✓ PINEAL GLAND

- ✓ PITUITARY GLAND

- ✓ INTUITION

- ✓ CEREBROSPINAL FLUID

- ✓ CREATION IS BASED ON IONS GAIN AND LOSS OF ENERGY BASED ON ELECTRONS. ENERGY OR ELECTRICITY IS BASED ON NEGATIVE CHARGE

- ✓ CYANOBACTERIA

THE BOOK OF SELF A THESIS ON
ENERGY AND HOW IT INTERRELATES
FLOYD WILLIAMS

THE BOOK OF SELF A THESIS ON
ENERGY AND HOW IT INTERRELATES
FLOYD WILLIAMS

THE BOOK OF SELF A THESIS ON
ENERGY AND HOW IT INTERRELATES
FLOYD WILLIAMS

THE BOOK OF SELF A THESIS OF
ENERGY AND HOW IT INTERRELATES
FLOYD WILLIAMS

THE BOOK OF SELF A THESIS ON
ENERGY AND HOW IT INTERRELATES
FLOYD WILLIAMS

THE BOOK OF SELF A THESIS ON
ENERGY AND HOW IT INTERRELATES
FLOYD WILLIAMS

THE BOOK OF SELF A THESIS ON
ENERGY AND HOW IT INTERRELATES
FLOYD WILLIAMS